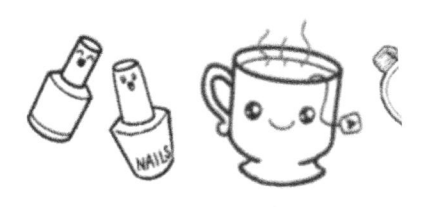

This Book Belongs To

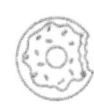

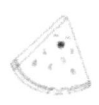

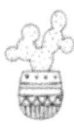

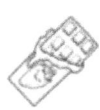

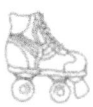

_____

*I recommend using pencil, colored pencil or gel pens to reduce bleed through when coloring in this book.

*This book is designed to keep track of your period and your PMS symptoms for one year as well as provide pages for reflection, journaling and fun art practice.

*Your period is a normal, natural and heathy occurance.
*If you track your period every month, you may notice a pattern. It may become easier to tell when you will get your next period and you may discover things that help alleviate any discomforts.
*A menstrual cycle is counted from the first day of bleeding in one month to the first day of bleeding in the next month.
*The average menstrual cycle is about 28 days, but cycles that are 21-45 days are also normal. It may take 6 years or more after your period starts for your cycle to become regular.

Please enjoy and provide feedback so I can create to best journals and Trackers for my customers.

Copyright 2020
Moon Time press

SOME COMMON TYPES OF PERIOD PRODUCTS

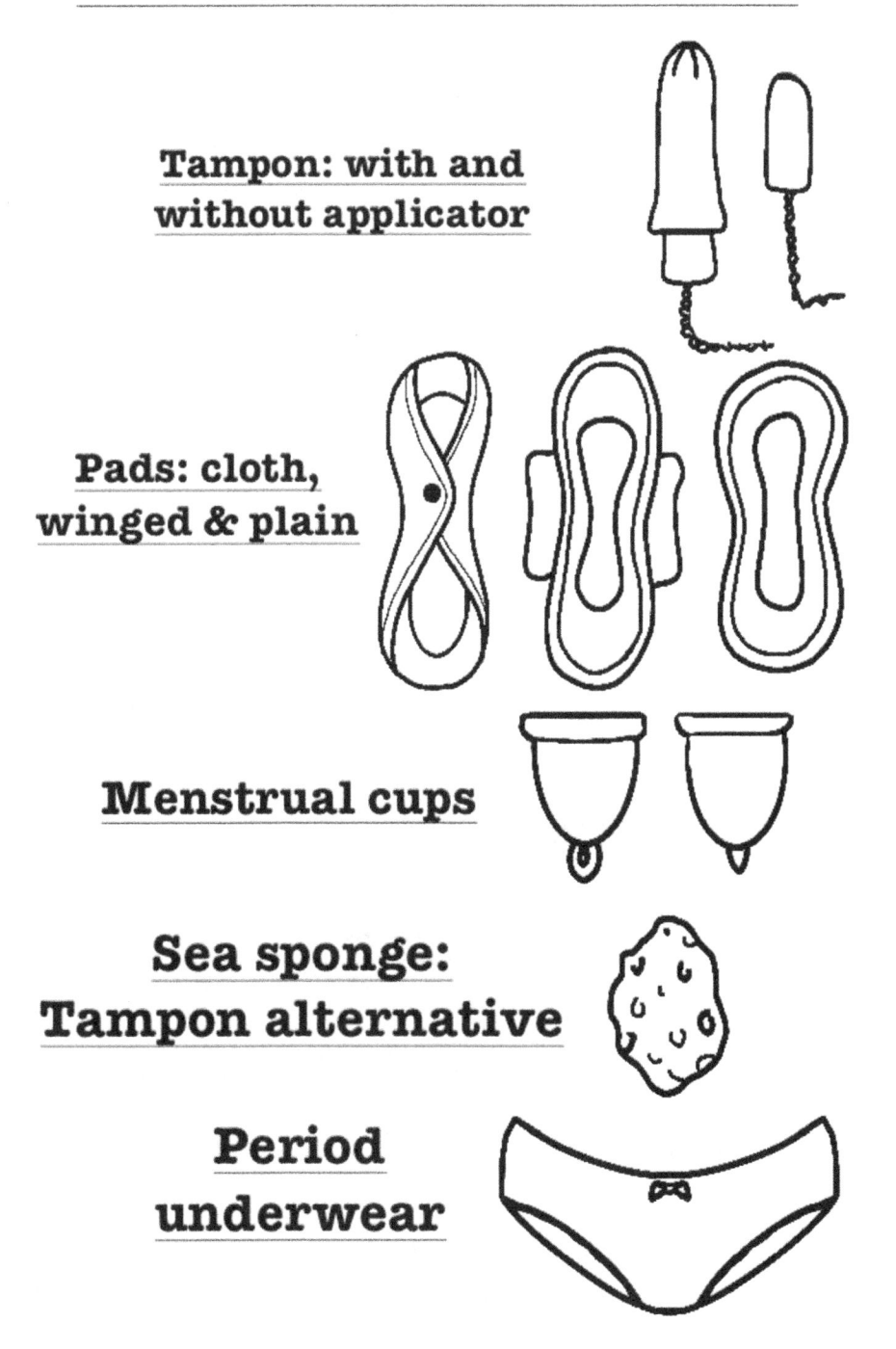

Tampon: with and without applicator

Pads: cloth, winged & plain

Menstrual cups

Sea sponge: Tampon alternative

Period underwear

Female Reproductive System

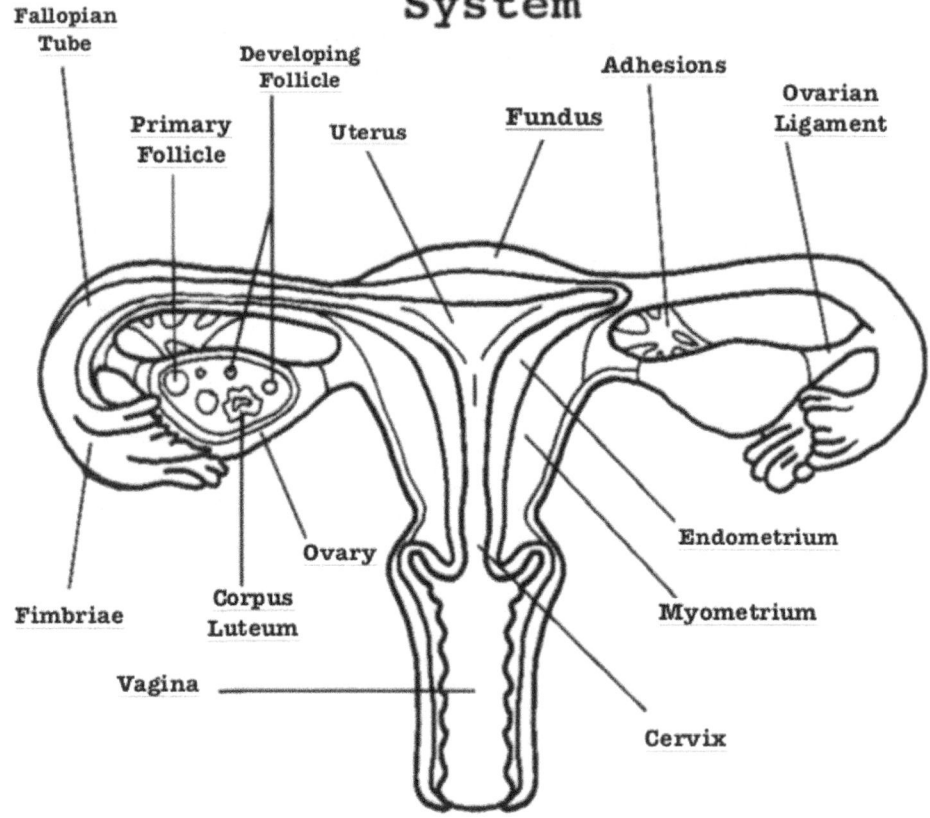

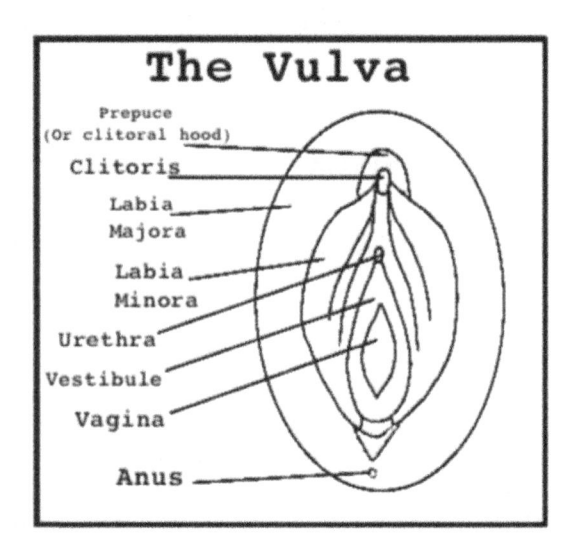

- Fallopian Tube
- Primary Follicle
- Developing Follicle
- Uterus
- Fundus
- Adhesions
- Ovarian Ligament
- Fimbriae
- Ovary
- Corpus Luteum
- Vagina
- Endometrium
- Myometrium
- Cervix

The Vulva

- Prepuce (Or clitoral hood)
- Clitoris
- Labia Majora
- Labia Minora
- Urethra
- Vestibule
- Vagina
- Anus

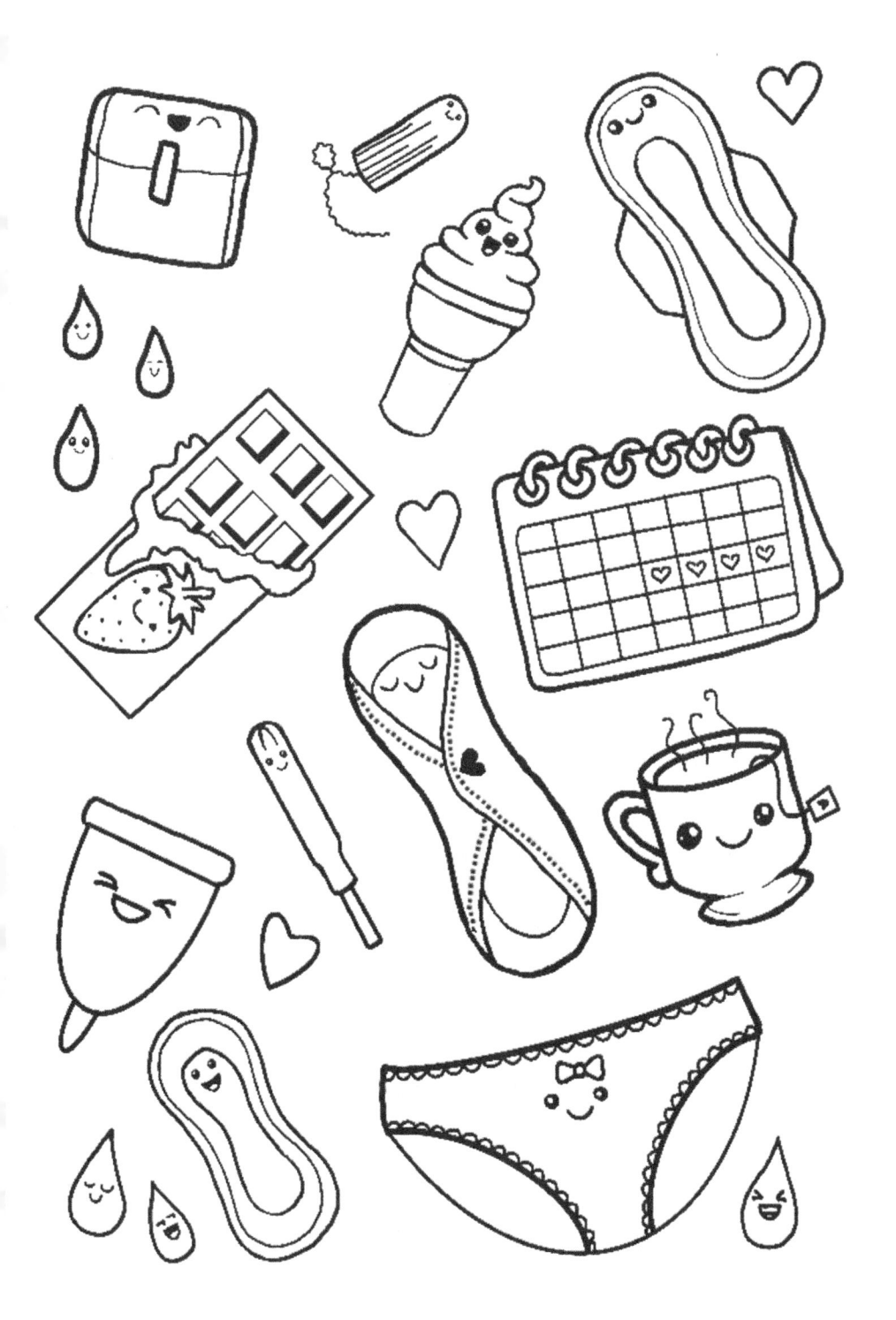

Month: _____   Year: _____

Sun	Mon	Tue	Wed	Thurs	Fri	Sat

days since last period ☐

○ light
○○ medium
○○○ heavy

next period expected date ☐

Mark the days you have your period on the calendar. You can mark them using the flow key or draw hearts, stars or anything you like.

PMS symptoms

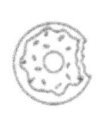

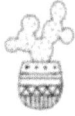

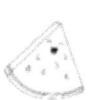

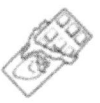

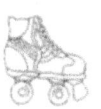

Write down anything you may be experiencing during your period. Include your moods, any cravings, aches, cramps or tenderness you are feeling and anything you did that helped.

Day 1	
Day 2	
Day 3	
Day 4	
Day 5	
Day 6	
Day 7	

Notes:

① ② ③ ④

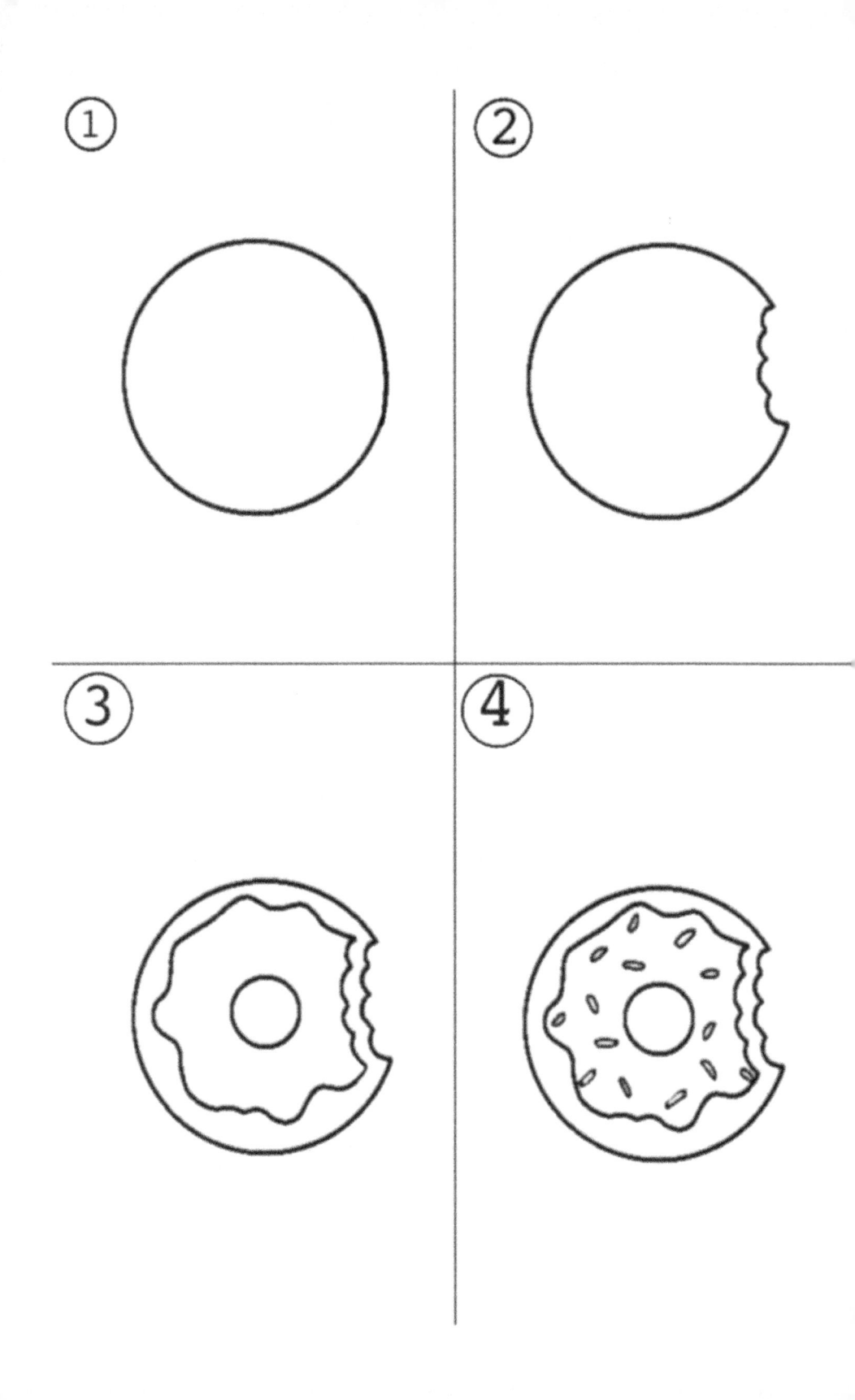

Month: _____ Year: _____

	Sun	Mon	Tue	Wed	Thurs	Fri	Sat

days since last period ☐

next period expected date ☐

○ light
○○ medium
○○○ heavy

Mark the days you have your period on the calendar. You can mark them using the flow key or draw hearts, stars or anything you like.

PMS symptoms

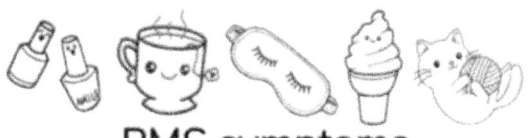

Write down anything you may be experiencing during your period. Include your moods, any cravings, aches, cramps or tenderness you are feeling and anything you did that helped.

Day 1	
Day 2	
Day 3	
Day 4	
Day 5	
Day 6	
Day 7	

Notes:

① ② ③ ④

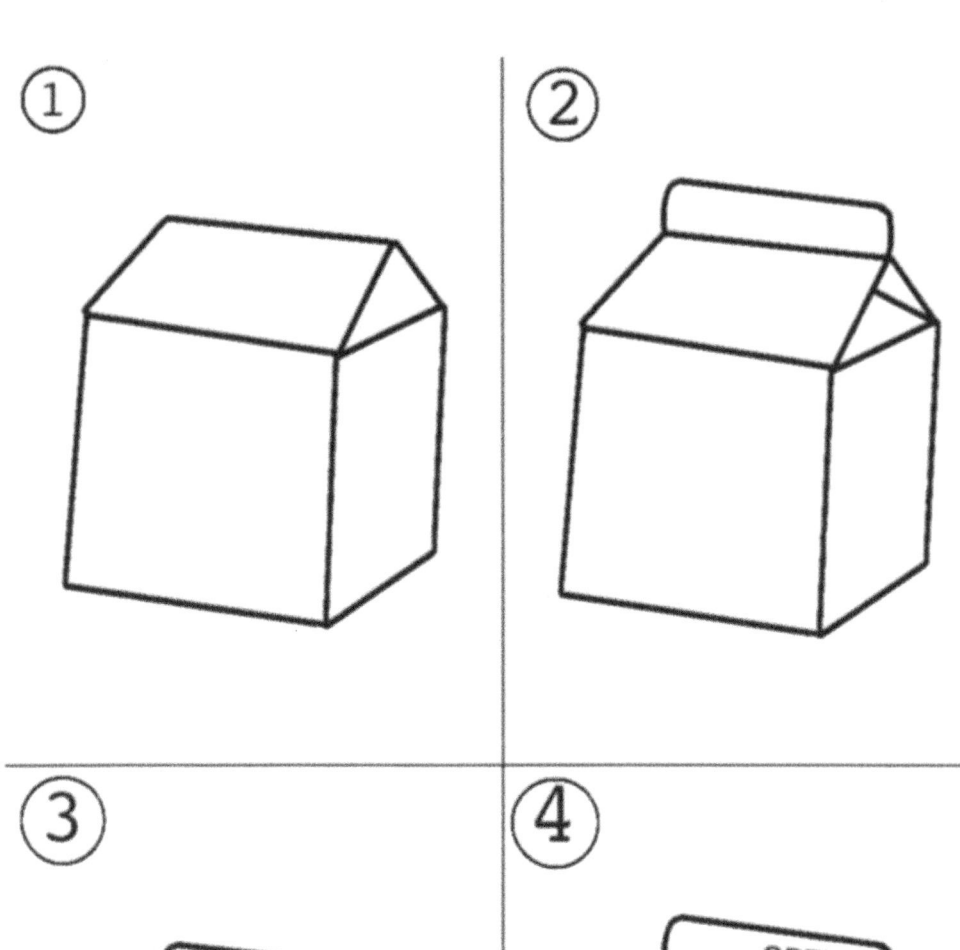

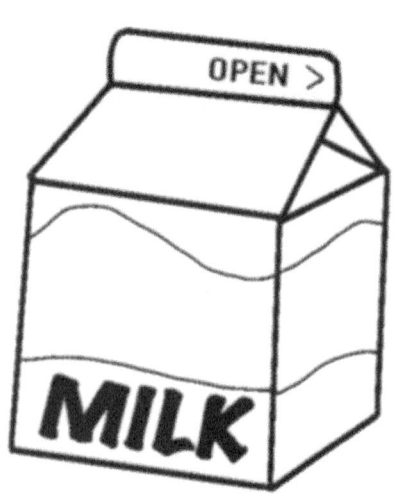

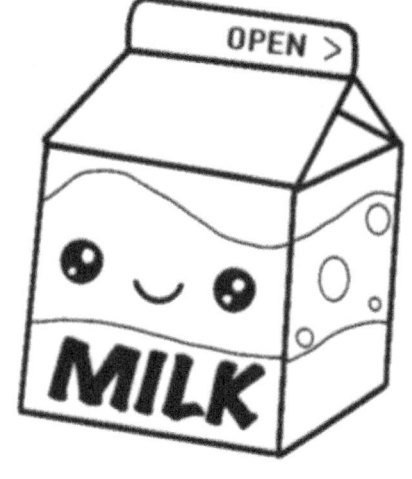

OPEN >
MILK

Month: _____   Year: _____

Sun	Mon	Tue	Wed	Thurs	Fri	Sat

days since last period ☐

next period expected date ☐

○ light
○○ medium
○○○ heavy

Mark the days you have your period on the calendar. You can mark them using the flow key or draw hearts, stars or anything you like.

PMS symptoms

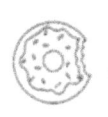

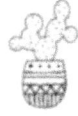

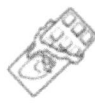

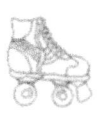

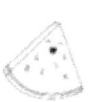

Write down anything you may be experiencing during your period. Include your moods, any cravings, aches, cramps or tenderness you are feeling and anything you did that helped.

Day 1	
Day 2	
Day 3	
Day 4	
Day 5	
Day 6	
Day 7	

Notes:

① ② ③ ④

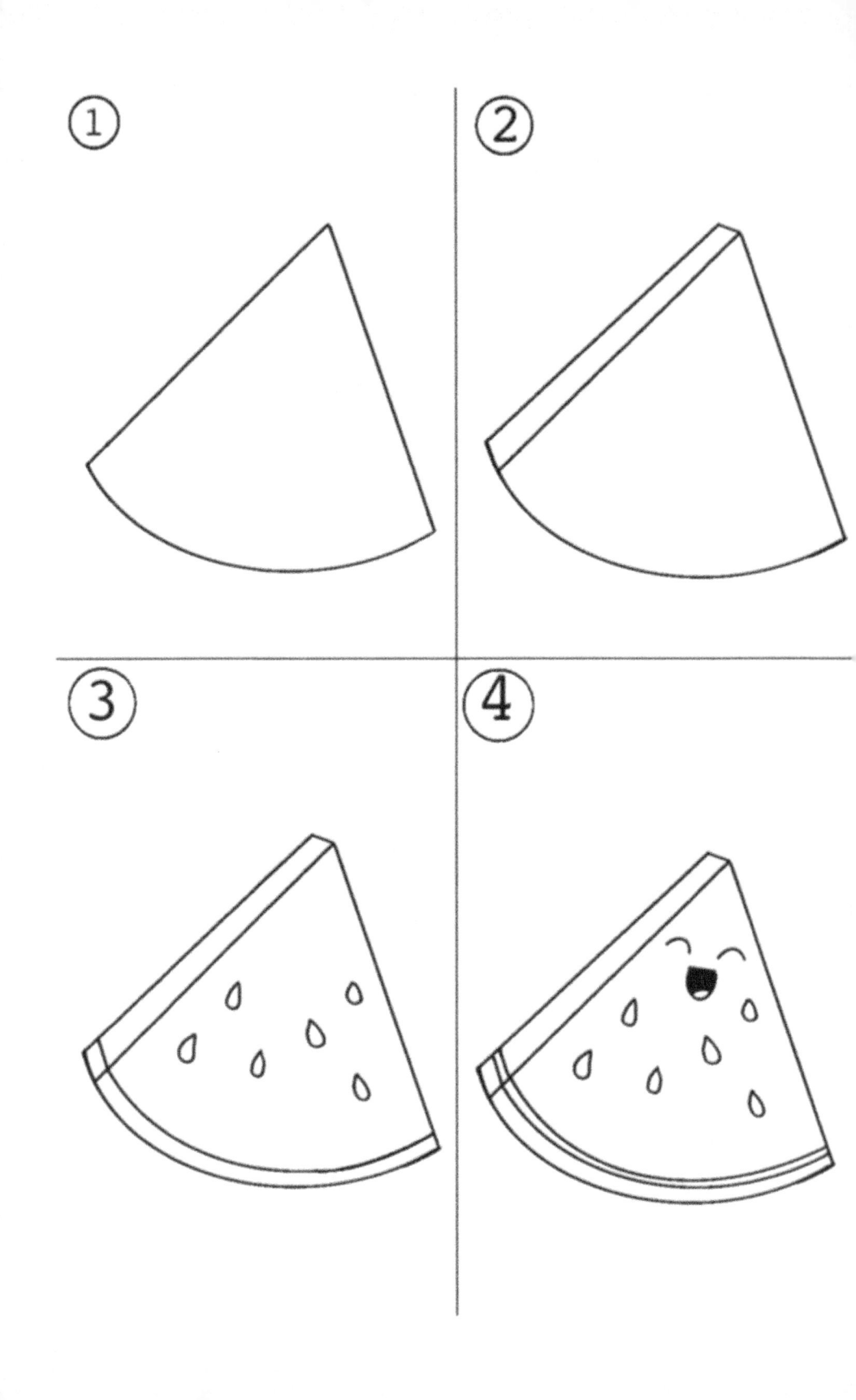

Month: Year:

Sun	Mon	Tue	Wed	Thurs	Fri	Sat

days since last period

○ light
○○ medium
○○○ heavy

next period expected date

Mark the days you have your period on the calendar. You can mark them using the flow key or draw hearts, stars or anything you like.

PMS symptoms

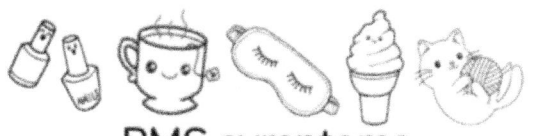

Write down anything you may be experiencing during your period. Include your moods, any cravings, aches, cramps or tenderness you are feeling and anything you did that helped.

Day 1	
Day 2	
Day 3	
Day 4	
Day 5	
Day 6	
Day 7	

Notes:

① ② ③ ④

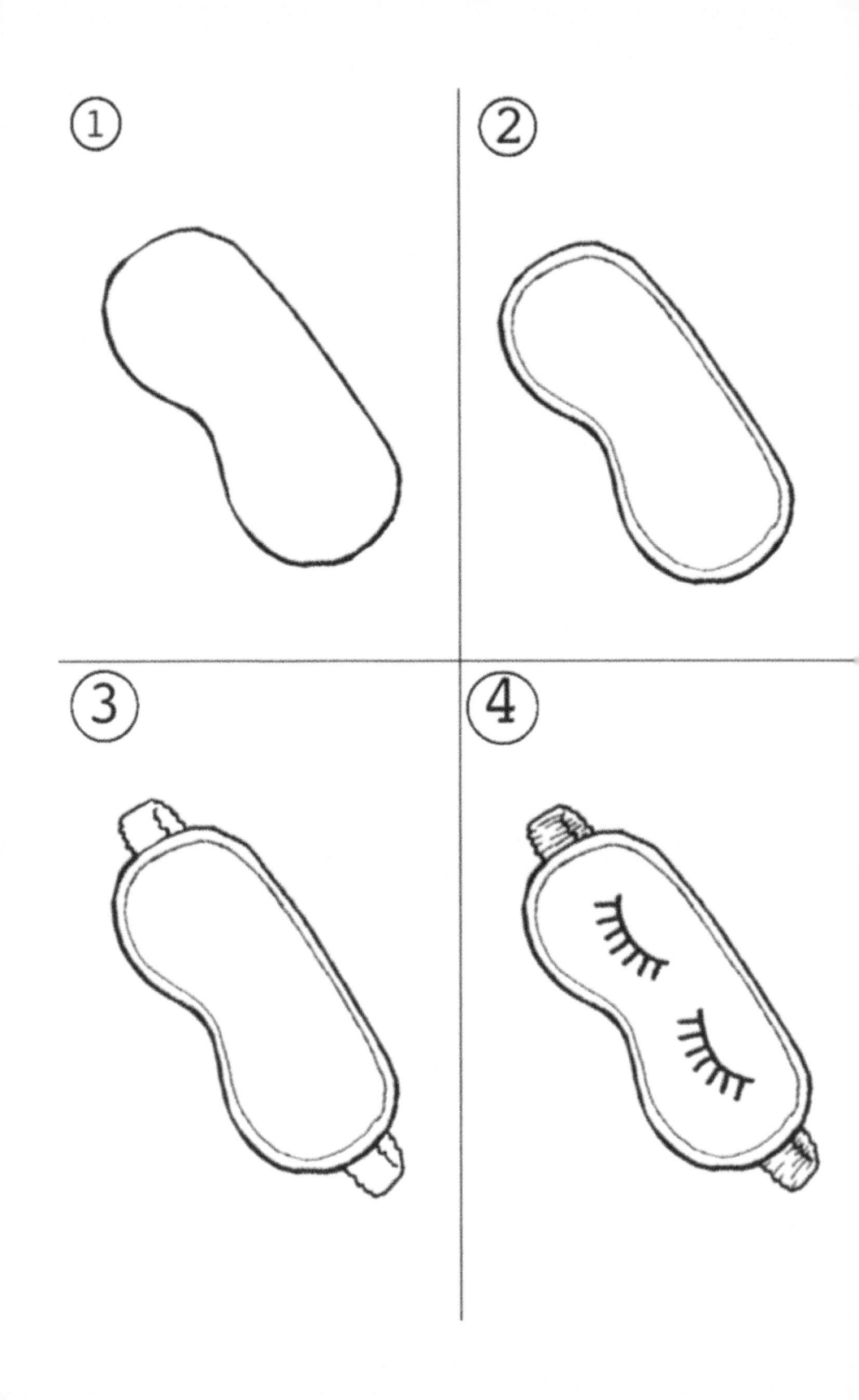

Month: _____   Year: _____

Sun	Mon	Tue	Wed	Thurs	Fri	Sat

days since last period ☐

next period expected date ☐

◊ light
◊◊ medium
◊◊◊ heavy

Mark the days you have your period on the calendar. You can mark them using the flow key or draw hearts, stars or anything you like.

PMS symptoms

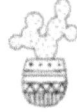

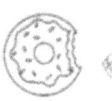

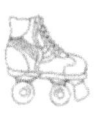

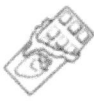

Write down anything you may be experiencing during your period. Include your moods, any cravings, aches, cramps or tenderness you are feeling and anything you did that helped.

Day 1	
Day 2	
Day 3	
Day 4	
Day 5	
Day 6	
Day 7	

Notes:

① ② ③ ④

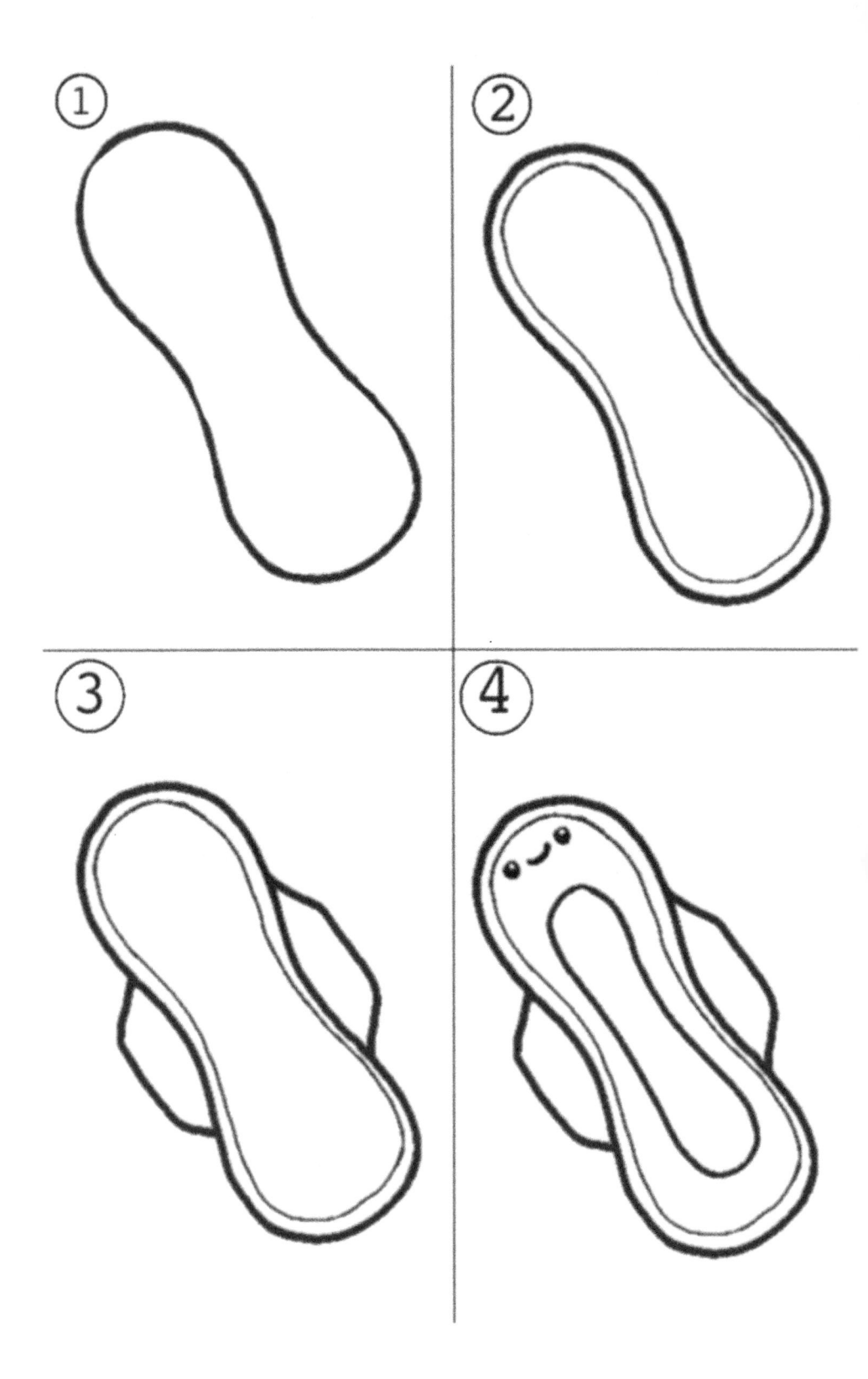

Month: Year:

Sun	Mon	Tue	Wed	Thurs	Fri	Sat

days since last period

next period expected date

light
medium
heavy

Mark the days you have your period on the calendar. You can mark them using the flow key or draw hearts, stars or anything you like.

PMS symptoms

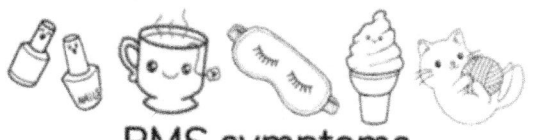

Write down anything you may be experiencing during your period. Include your moods, any cravings, aches, cramps or tenderness you are feeling and anything you did that helped.

Day 1	
Day 2	
Day 3	
Day 4	
Day 5	
Day 6	
Day 7	

Notes:

① ② ③ ④

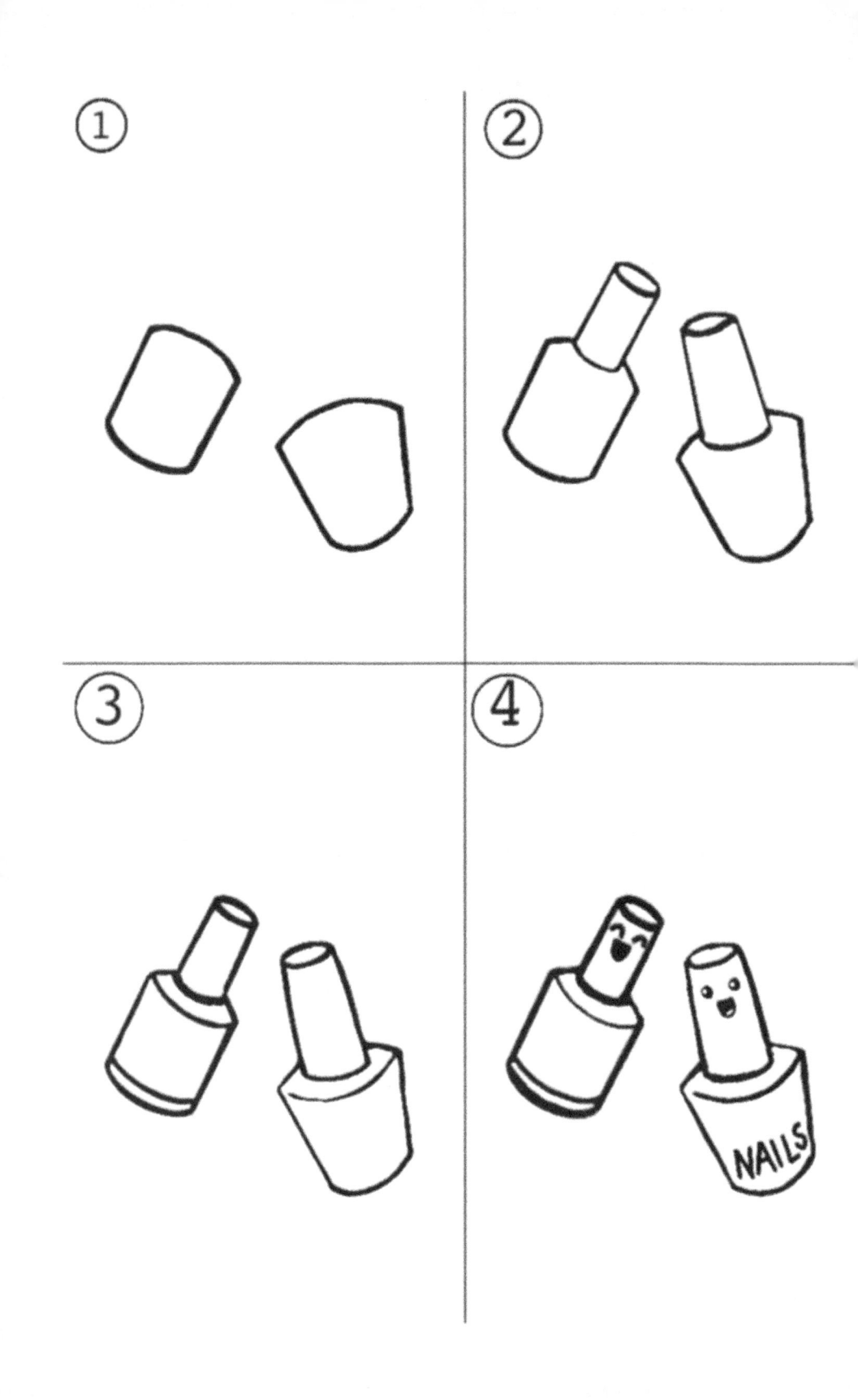

Month: _____   Year: _____

Sun	Mon	Tue	Wed	Thurs	Fri	Sat

◊ light
◊ ◊ medium
◊ ◊ ◊ heavy

days since last period ☐

next period expected date ☐

Mark the days you have your period on the calendar. You can mark them using the flow key or draw hearts, stars or anything you like.

PMS symptoms

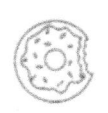

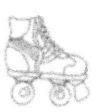

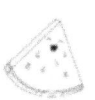

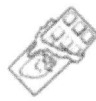

Write down anything you may be experiencing during your period. Include your moods, any cravings, aches, cramps or tenderness you are feeling and anything you did that helped.

Day 1	
Day 2	
Day 3	
Day 4	
Day 5	
Day 6	
Day 7	

Notes:

① ② ③ ④

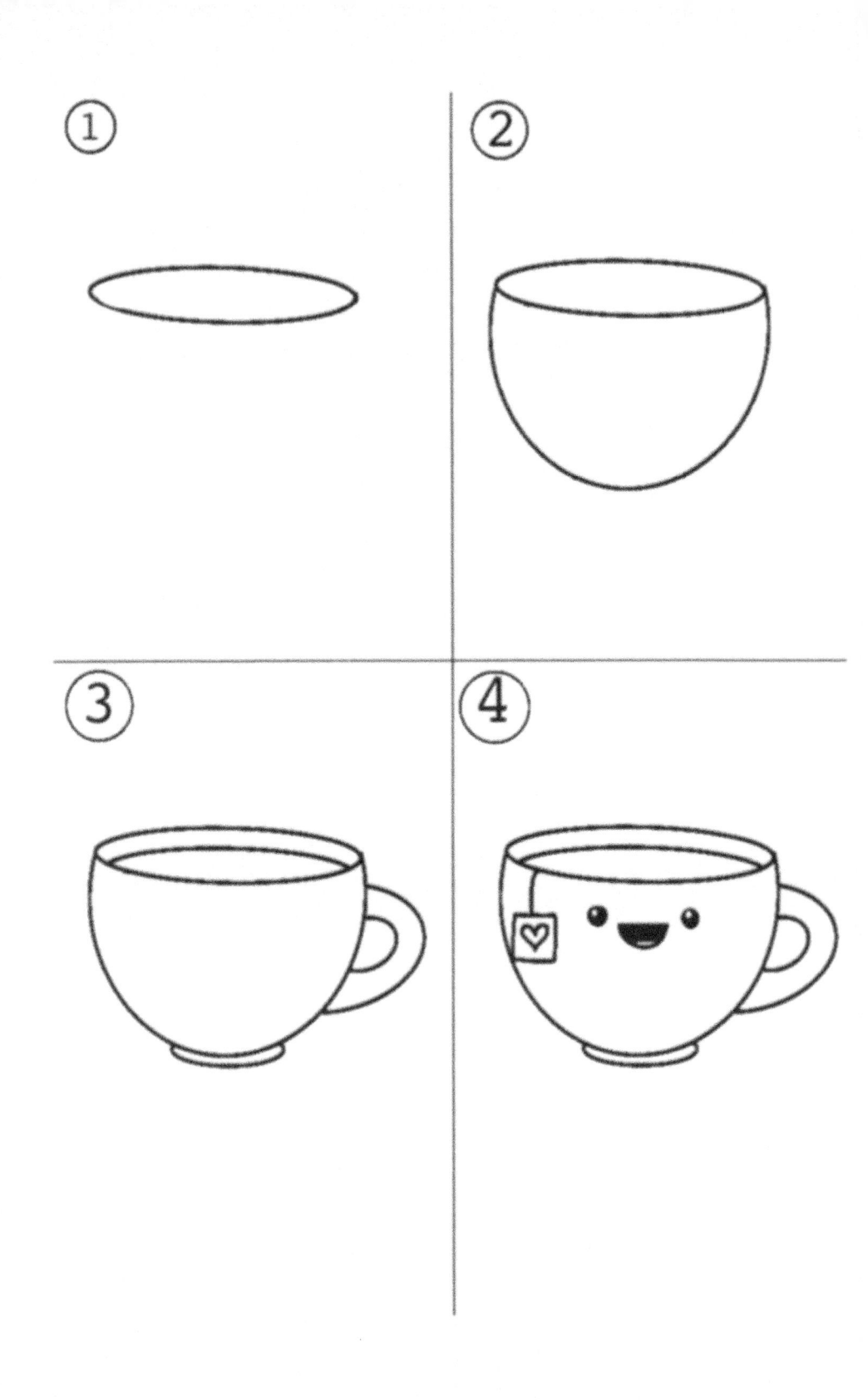

Month: _____ Year: _____

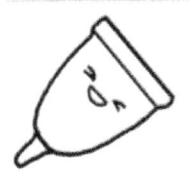

Sun	Mon	Tue	Wed	Thurs	Fri	Sat

days since last period ☐

next period expected date ☐

◌ light
◌ ◌ medium
◌ ◌ ◌ heavy

Mark the days you have your period on the calendar. You can mark them using the flow key or draw hearts, stars or anything you like.

PMS symptoms

Write down anything you may be experiencing during your period. Include your moods, any cravings, aches, cramps or tenderness you are feeling and anything you did that helped.

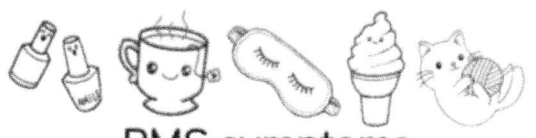

Day 1	
Day 2	
Day 3	
Day 4	
Day 5	
Day 6	
Day 7	

Notes:

① ② ③ ④

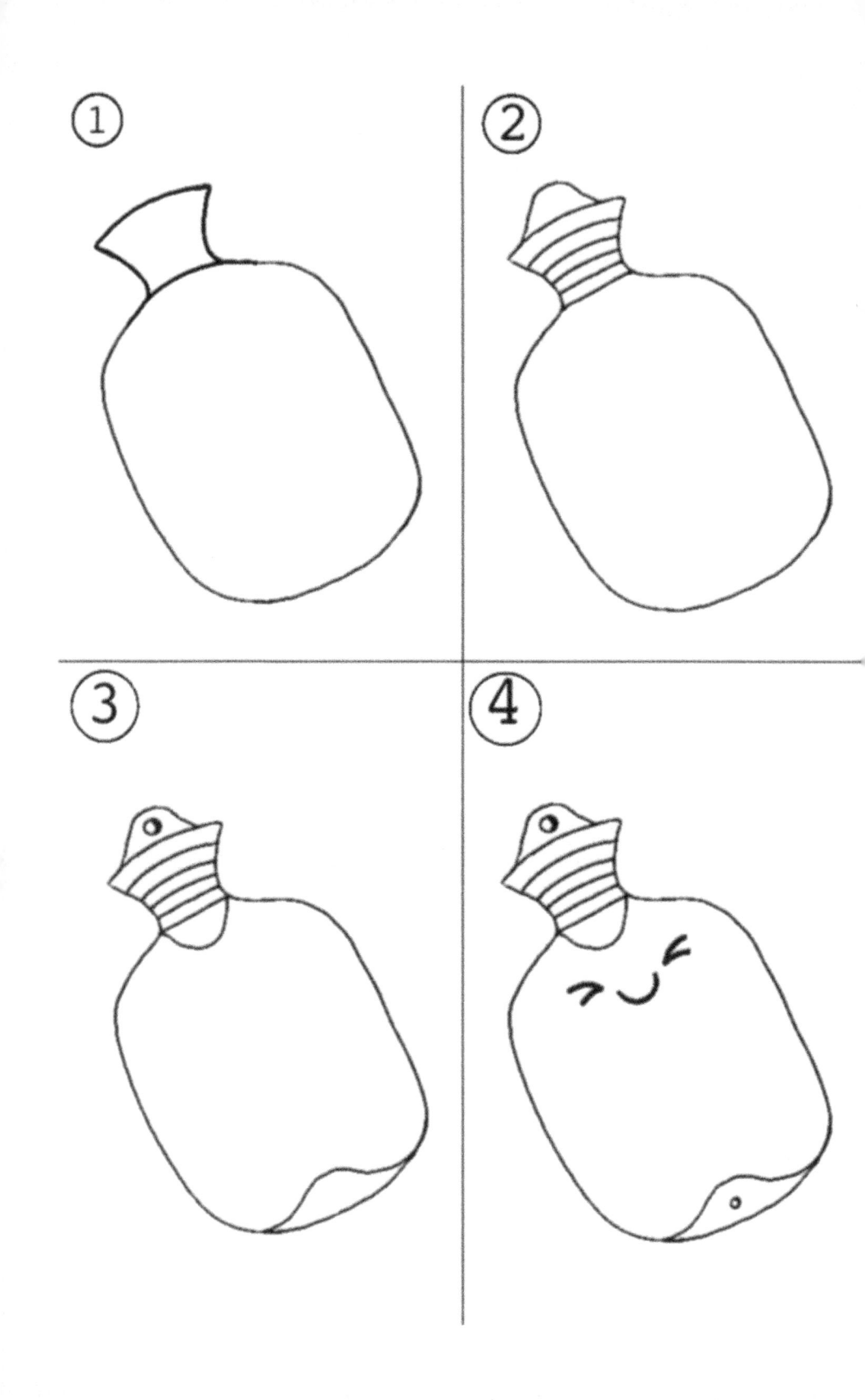

Month: _____   Year: _____

Sun	Mon	Tue	Wed	Thurs	Fri	Sat

△ light
△△ medium
△△△ heavy

days since last period ☐

next period expected date ☐

Mark the days you have your period on the calendar. You can mark them using the flow key or draw hearts, stars or anything you like.

PMS symptoms

Write down anything you may be experiencing during your period. Include your moods, any cravings, aches, cramps or tenderness you are feeling and anything you did that helped.

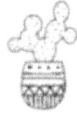

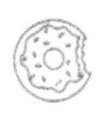

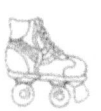

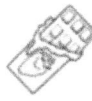

Day 1	
Day 2	
Day 3	
Day 4	
Day 5	
Day 6	
Day 7	

Notes:

① ② ③ ④

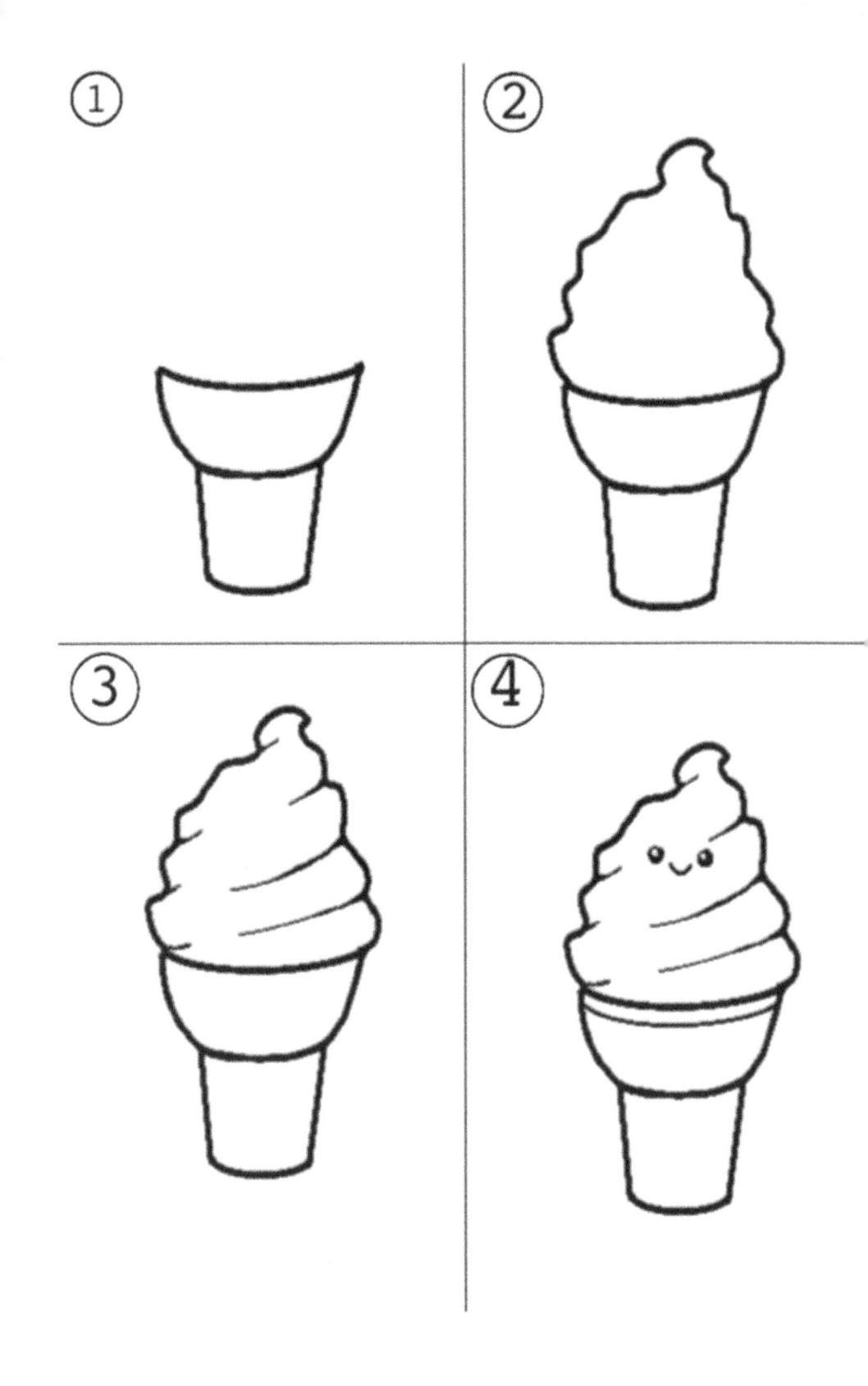

Month: _____ Year: _____

Sun	Mon	Tue	Wed	Thurs	Fri	Sat

○ light
○○ medium
○○○ heavy

days since last period ☐

next period expected date ☐

Mark the days you have your period on the calendar. You can mark them using the flow key or draw hearts, stars or anything you like.

PMS symptoms

Write down anything you may be experiencing during your period. Include your moods, any cravings, aches, cramps or tenderness you are feeling and anything you did that helped.

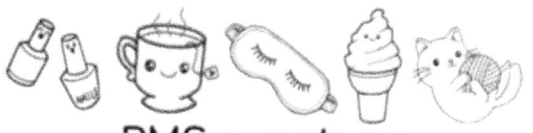

Day 1	
Day 2	
Day 3	
Day 4	
Day 5	
Day 6	
Day 7	

Notes:

① ② ③ ④

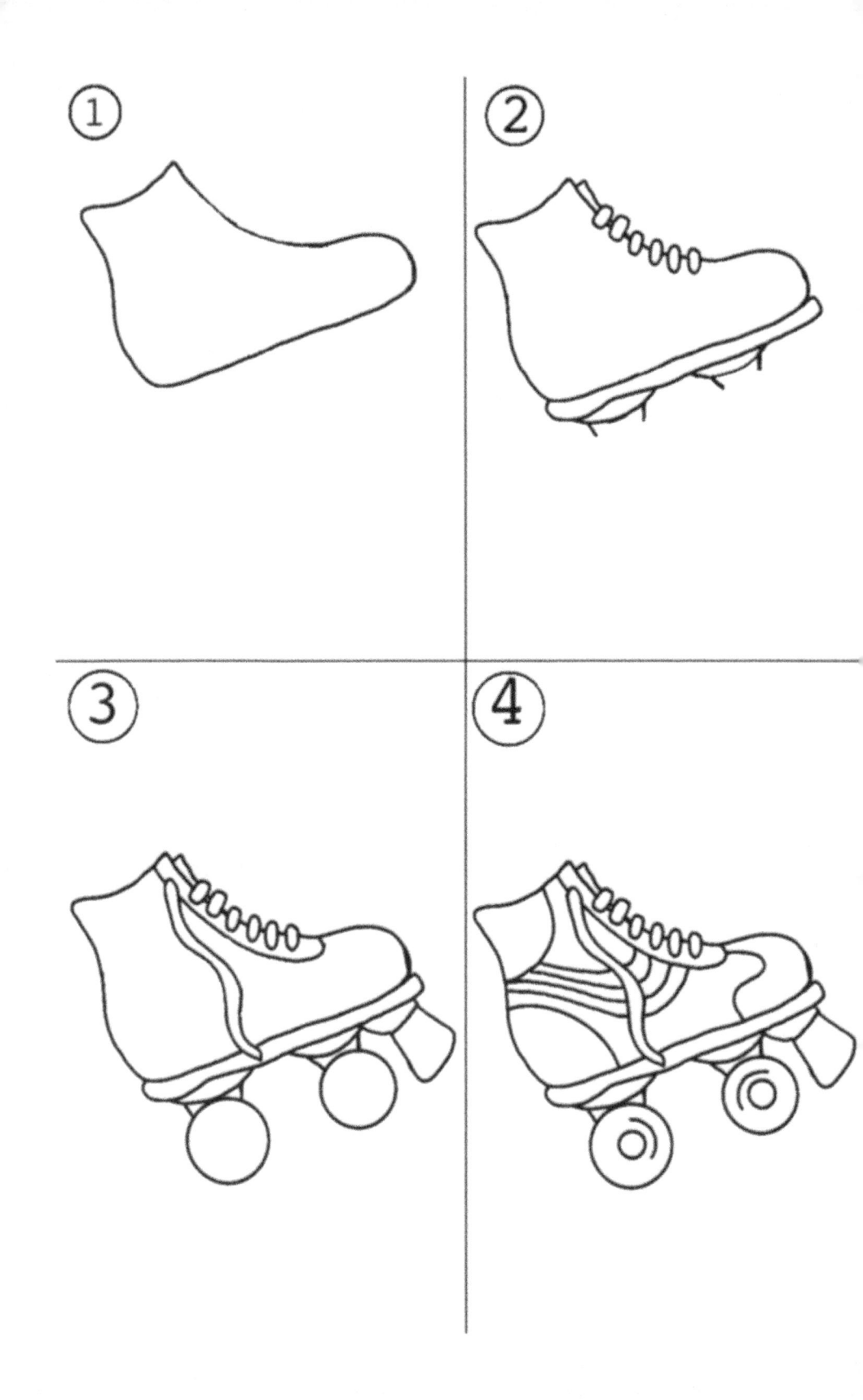

Month: _____ Year: _____

Sun	Mon	Tue	Wed	Thurs	Fri	Sat

days since last period ☐

next period expected date ☐

○ light
○○ medium
○○○ heavy

Mark the days you have your period on the calendar. You can mark them using the flow key or draw hearts, stars or anything you like.

PMS symptoms

Write down anything you may be experiencing during your period. Include your moods, any cravings, aches, cramps or tenderness you are feeling and anything you did that helped.

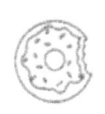

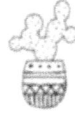

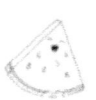

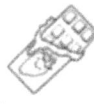

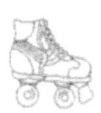

Day 1	
Day 2	
Day 3	
Day 4	
Day 5	
Day 6	
Day 7	

Notes:

① ② ③ ④

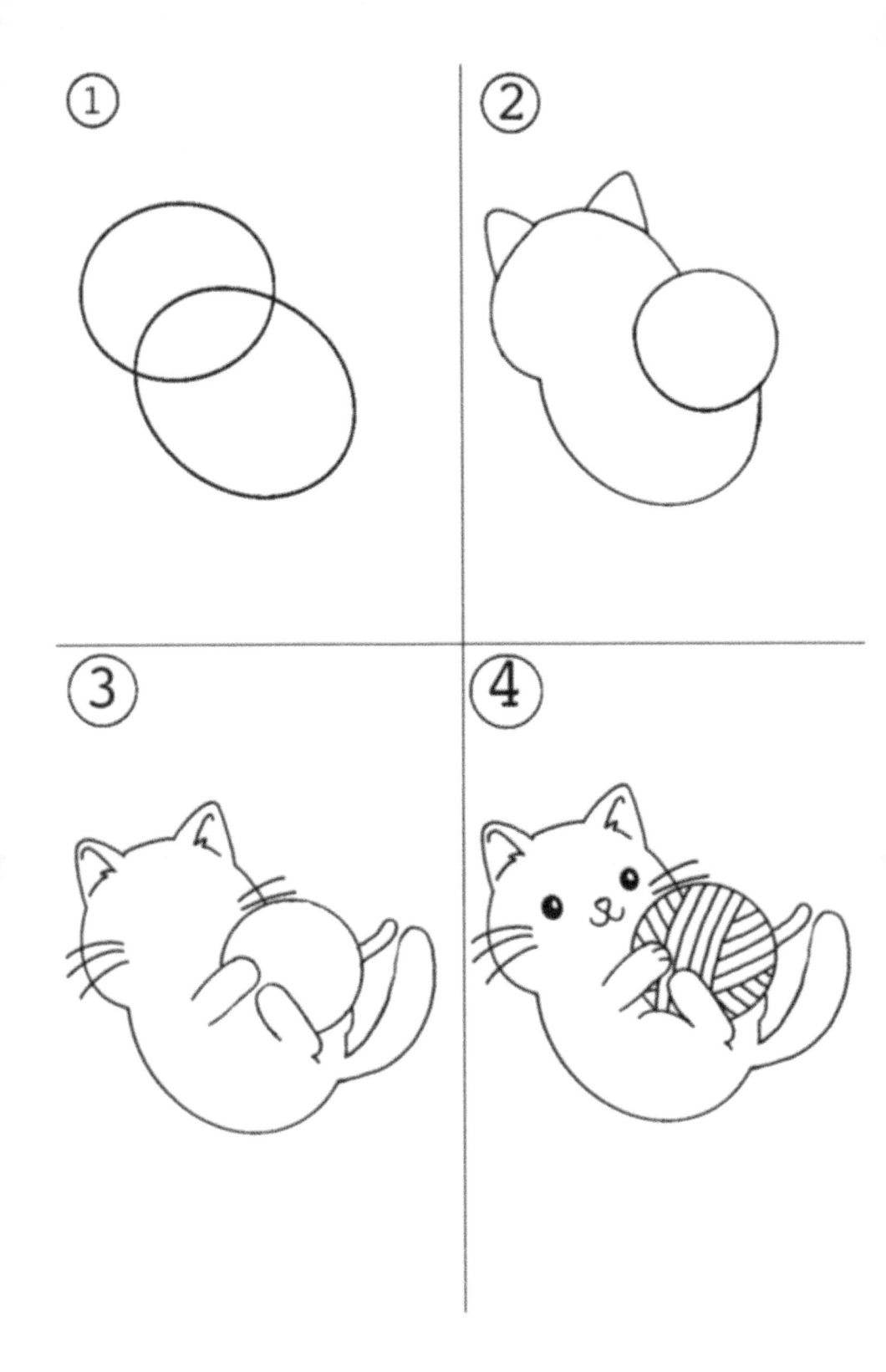

Month: _____   Year: _____

Sun	Mon	Tue	Wed	Thurs	Fri	Sat

○ light
○○ medium
○○○ heavy

days since last period ☐

next period expected date ☐

Mark the days you have your period on the calendar. You can mark them using the flow key or draw hearts, stars or anything you like.

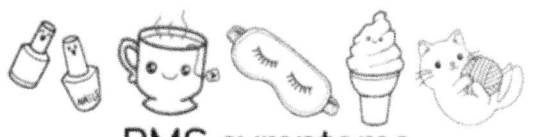

PMS symptoms

Write down anything you may be experiencing during your period. Include your moods, any cravings, aches, cramps or tenderness you are feeling and anything you did that helped.

Day 1	
Day 2	
Day 3	
Day 4	
Day 5	
Day 6	
Day 7	

Notes:

① ② ③ ④

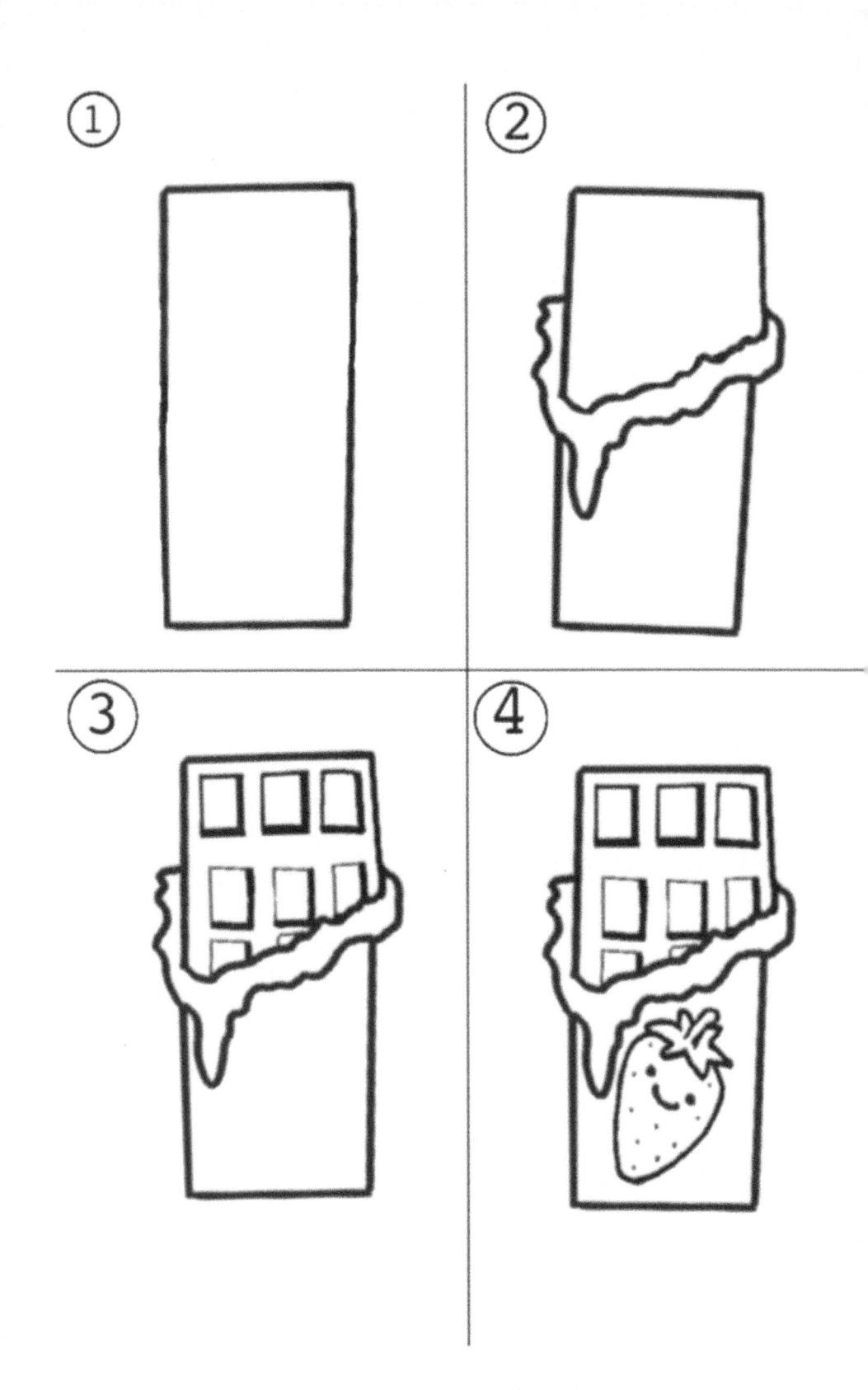

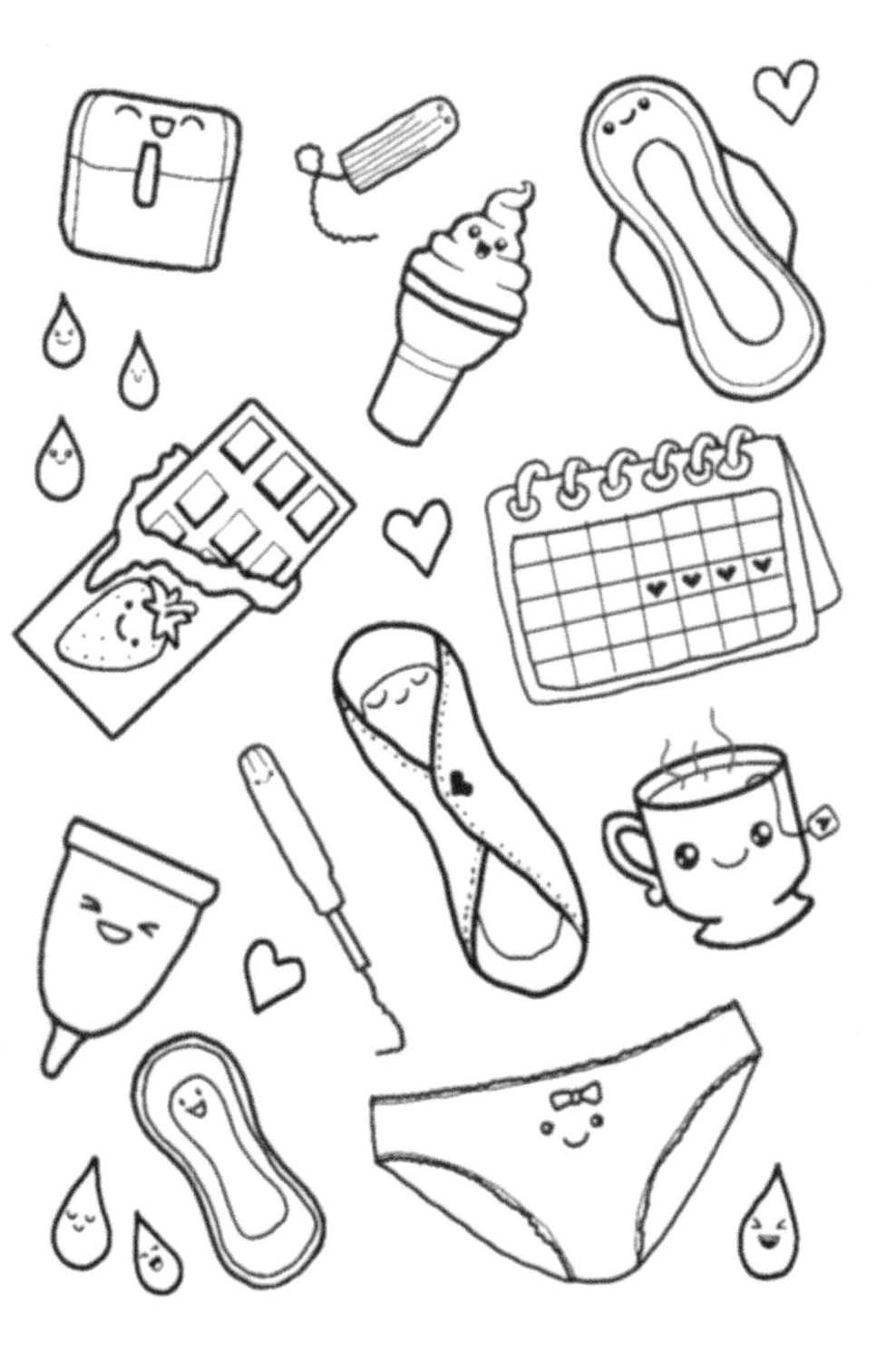

Made in the USA
Las Vegas, NV
05 July 2025